The #AskDrA Book

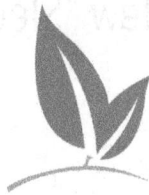

Dr. Guillermo Alvarez

Rob Anspach

The #AskDrA Book

Easy & Practical Answers
To Enjoying Life
As A New "Sleever".

*Based On The First 26 Episodes Of The #AskDrA Show.

The #AskDrA Book

Published by: Anspach Media
P.O. Box 2
Conestoga Pa 17516

ISBN 10: 0-9894663-3-7

ISBN 13: 978-0-9894663-3-2

While they have made every effort to verify the information provided in this publication, neither the author(s) nor the publisher assumes any responsibility for errors in, omissions from or different interpretation of the subject matter.

The information herein may be subject to varying laws and practices in different areas, states and countries. The reader assumes all responsibility for use of the information.

** *Disclaimer: Individual results may vary. The statements on this website and all affiliates have not been evaluated by the FDA. Products mentioned on this website are not intended to diagnose, treat, cure or prevent any disease and do not replace medical advice. Advice on treatment or care of an individual patient should be obtained through consultation with a physician or trained health care practitioner who has examined that patient or is familiar with that patient's medical history.*

Dedicated

To my patients for showing me and teaching me more than I ever expected. To my teammates for jumping on board with me in this crusade to help out people worldwide struggling with obesity.

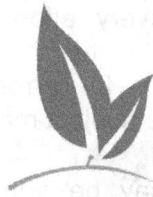

Contents

Contents Continued...

Forward

By: Rob Anspach

I just have to say, "WOW"! I remember going back and forth on Facebook chat with Dr. Alvarez in May 2015 on what the name of the new show would be and what it would cover. Then being in his backyard two months later while Episode 3 of the #AskDrA Show was being filmed, felt very surreal.

Now this book! It's just incredible the journey this one idea has become. Let's forget, just for a moment, that you have an incredible resource guide in front of you, that's designed to help you stay focused on your health after getting a sleeve...and let me share with you my story of visiting Dr. A face to face for the very first time.

I had never been to Mexico before, and frankly never even heard of Piedras Negras prior to becoming friends with Dr. Alvarez. And, yes, I had the same questions that his over 10,000 patients have had. I was anxious about the whole crossing the border thing, I was wondering about the crime they talk about on TV, I was worried about eating the food or drinking the water and I was concerned about my safety.

Funny thing was, as many questions as I had, Dr. A was more than willing to answer them all. It was like I was his only focus at that moment. That speaks volumes to me...about his character, about how he treats his patients, about his work ethic and his dedication to his family, friends and patients.

My wife and I had the privilege of meeting his staff, his father and his wife. All great people. Every single one of them. They all made us feel safe. Like we were part of the family.

The moment we entered his office, Dr. A. was there greeting us with a handshake, a smile and a hug. And although we weren't there for surgery, I could tell he treated all his patients and visitors with care and respect.

Yes, he's truly the real deal…the same person you see on his videos, that shares answers to patient submitted questions, that acts silly sometimes, is the same person that greets you when you arrive.

What I really like is that he's big on educating his patients. He truly wants to change their lives, to give them a second chance and to help them improve their overall health. He does this by constantly blogging, posting to social media, creating YouTube and Facebook videos, tweeting, and getting fans to engage him on Snapchat. Something most American doctors don't even do.

So, now you know a little bit about how this book came to be, who Dr. A is and what makes him a fantastic choice for your weight loss surgery.

Enjoy the book!

Introduction

By: Dr. Guillermo Alvarez

All throughout my professional life, my goal has been to pass as much information onto my patients as possible. I truly believe that knowledge is power and that knowing more about your body and what to expect before and after your surgery gives you the tools to get more out of your procedure.

I started with old traditional ways like flyers, brochures, then moved up to emails. I even tried a radio program for over a year called Obesity Chat. It was a great start but I noticed that once the program ended patients were not able to recover that information given on that show. Then I thought of recording these episodes and creating a podcast. Unfortunately, patients were not that into podcasts or downloading episodes or streaming to their devices.

That was when I turned to YouTube. I thought "What a great idea! Not only can I do the show but it will be there for future use. Patients can then use it as a reference and even go back to a particular episode looking for a specific answer." So that's how The #AskDrA Show was born.

The goal was all about content. Of course, as we advanced with each show we started improving it with better lighting, crisper sound, smoother editing and even video clips from actual fans and patients.

The show is aired weekly no matter where I am, whether at a conference, in the hospital, or even on vacation. The show is posted to YouTube then distributed and shared on social media networks, obesity websites, blogs, newsletters and even fans and patients share it via text and chat.

This brings a big smile to my face to be able to help so many people who did not have the good fortune to have a surgical team, doctor or group that was accessible to their questions. My team and I support absolutely anyone who is in need or is searching for information trying to get more out of their surgery.

We wanted to bring the essence of the show to print. The idea is for you to have a reference of questions and answers, a place to turn to, a source of information that you can use before and/or after surgery. You'll notice as you read along that we packed into this book a lot of questions (over two dozen shows worth). But, always keep in mind that if you don't find an answer to a question you can always reach out to me by using the hashtag #AskDrA and I'll be there for you.

I hope you enjoy the book but most importantly that it brings you knowledge.

Dr. Alvarez

P.S. Follow along by using the links on each chapter to watch the corresponding #AskDrA Show episode.

Chapter 1

Gurgling, Vitamins, Proteins & Superfoods

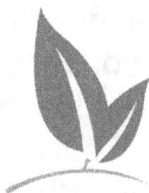

"Don't get overwhelmed with the protein thing after weight loss surgery. It's not as hard as you may think."

To watch the #AskDrA Show episode that this chapter is based on, follow along at: www.bit.ly/AskDrA1

Is it normal to have gurgling in the throat, burning in the throat and ears 9 months out from sleeve?

The gurgling sensation, that noise or that feeling that you hear, feel, or even notice is a sign that the sleeve is swollen. My suggestion is to do a round of antacids for 10 to 15 days, 21 days if needed, and that gurgling sensation will go away. It's very important you redo these antacids every once in a while when you have that gurgling sensation or you hear the gurgling sounds. Because it's just a noise that is produced when liquid or food goes down into your sleeve. It's like pouring a lot of water into a funnel you'll hear that gurgling noise. It's normal. Expect that! Even if you're overly concerned and you go through the endoscopy process in most cases it all comes out normal, that means everything is fine. It's just that the swollen tissue of the sleeve is present. Make sure you take your antacids and take care of that sleeve.

If all your levels are good, do you still need to take vitamins daily?

Yes, even though your vitamin levels are good you should still take them. I recommend a multivitamin every day. I even take them. I don't have a sleeve but it's very important that you supplement your diet and nutritional needs with vitamins and minerals to make sure everything is good. Now, maybe down the road taking a vitamin is a hassle or you get tired of it. You can switch brands. You can switch the form. You can even do sublingual (under the tongue) B12. You can even do shots, if you don't like taking vitamins every once in a while. You can switch from the solid pills to the gummies. Work around this and take your multivitamins, take your vitamins, your supplements. They're very important!

What to buy before and after surgery to be prepared?

What to buy before surgery? That is a question that you'll have to touch base with your surgeon, or with your surgeon's team. That he or she will let you know what they prefer for you to buy. For us, we give our patients a shopping list that we recommend they have before coming for surgery. It includes the first week of liquids, all the recommendations we ask you to buy and also what to bring. Even though we ask you to pack lightly we do recommend that you have this shopping list and you go over it to make sure you have everything before coming here. If not using our service, I would touch base with your surgeon prior to having surgery and he or she will hopefully give you their list.

How long after surgery can one go to the chiropractor to get an adjustment?

Can you go to a chiropractor? Yes! But, I would recommend you wait at least fifteen days post op (after sleeve surgery). Don't worry, it doesn't mean that if you do get an adjustment with a chiropractor that something will move inside or burst your sleeve. I would recommend however, because of your incisions, to lay on your tummy. Or just wait until you feel comfortable and then you can go to the chiropractor.

What are your main go to protein sources as a vegan and would you recommend veganism to your patients?

It is very important for you to understand that protein just doesn't only come from meat. You can get protein from nuts, you can get them from kale, you can get them from mushrooms. All these are very good superfoods. People get overwhelmed with the protein thing after they have weight loss surgery. Just take it easy. It's not as hard as you may think, all right? Eating your veggies is a good source of protein maybe not as good of course as a piece of salmon or a lean steak. But you can make it through it easily being a vegan. We'll take a look at the super foods in a few minutes.

What procedure would you recommend, sleeve or band?

That's a good question, and I can go an hour just talking about the sleeve vs band. I would recommend the sleeve over the band anytime. The sleeve is a much better procedure than the band. I wouldn't even look at the band at all not anymore. We actually used to offer the band as a service, but removed it as a procedure about five years ago. We don't do them anymore. We do take bands out, though. And we do convert those bands into sleeves, but I wouldn't recommend a band nowadays. The sleeve is just better, no foreign body inside. You don't need any adjustments or any maintenance. Entrance of the stomach stays the same, the exit of the stomach stays the same. Hunger goes away with the sleeve not so much with the band.

Is there one "superfood" that you recommend I put into my diet?

There are some superfoods that are very important not only in a vegan's diet, but, of course, in any diet. And, you can make use of it too. Number 1... you can use kale, very important, very nutrient. Quinoa is also very good. And don't forget about Chia seeds. These types of super foods are highly recommended. They contain a lot of nutrients per serving that will benefit you. I use them a lot and once you get the hang of cooking them I'm sure you'll love them too.

How many calories per day should a gastric patient consume for better health and losing weight efficiency?

Normally after gastric sleeve surgery you will have the maximum point of restriction and will be limited to 600 to 800 calories per day. After about three to six months, you'll be up closer to 800 to 900 calories per month. Then about a year out you'll be consuming between 1,000 to 1,500 calories per day. Now those figures do vary slightly from patient to patient because of the size of the stomach. And, the size of a sleeve. And what size of bougie was used. If you stick to the numbers, your health will improve, your weight will drop off and your sleeve will stay happy.

Chapter 2

Dizziness, Sleeve Stretching, Restriction & Weight Gain

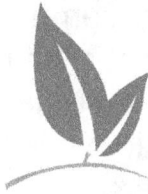

"It's very important when you decide to have a gastric sleeve you do get a sleeve with a surgeon that knows what he or she is doing!"

To watch the #AskDrA Show episode that this chapter is based on, follow along at:
www.bit.ly/AskDrA2

Can you stretch your sleeve over time back to the normal size stomach you had before?

The answer is, "no." There is just no way! If you had a correct and well done sleeve, there is no way you can actually stretch it out to the size of the stomach it used to be. What you can experience is that you are able to eat a little bit more. If you're comparing yourself to the first few months after your sleeve surgery where you're at the maximum point of restriction, then as the months go by that swollen sleeve tissue starts to come down, you're going to notice you're able to eat a bit more. It doesn't mean that you're stretching your sleeve, it means that the swollen tissue of the sleeve is healing.

Now, if you compare that amount of food that you're eating at that point to the first few weeks to months after your sleeve, yeah, it's going to be considerable. You might actually be doubling, or tripling the amount of food you're taking in, but is in no way comparable to the amount of food you were eating before surgery. Keep that in mind. If you're eating more, does it mean that you're eating more from before the surgery? Or are you eating more just compared to the first few weeks after surgery.

When I get full I feel light headed, also is it normal to still have dizzy spells 3 months post operation?

All right, let me explain...the dizziness or the dizzy spells are expected. They are normal. They are caused while you are going through that rapid weight loss phase. Usually lasts through the first eight to ten months or so. The dizziness or dizzy spells that people mention are common, they can be frequent, and if you decide to skip a meal, you're very likely to get them. If you skip two meals...you will get them. If you skip some carbs, you may get them. Be very careful not to skip a meal because you will be destined to have these dizzy spells or the dizziness.

It's important to schedule your meals. Do a balanced diet the first two or three months. It will help you avoid the dizziness. Some people even with all of that may still get them. It's important for you to understand that in certain situations, like moving very quickly, tying your shoe laces and getting up right away really quick, or getting up from bed may cause some dizziness. It's normal, it's expected, and it lasts just a few seconds, but it's a very small price to pay to be healthier and thinner.

I am 29 months out. I have no restriction. What should I do? I've gained 45 pounds within a year.

Let's talk about surgical technique. It is very important for you to understand that a well-crafted sleeve will give you the restriction you need. In this case, if you don't feel the restriction something may be wrong. You need to check with your doctor, your surgeon, to make sure you know how your sleeve was crafted. You should know about your sleeve. What the doctors experience was, how big your sleeve is, what bougie size did they decide to do on you, and what outcome should you expect down the road.

That is why it's very important when you decide to have gastric sleeve surgery, you get a sleeve from a surgeon that knows what he or she is doing, that they are certified, and that they have enough experience on this procedure. Because, although it may seem like it's a really simple procedure, and in most cases the actual surgery only takes about 30 minutes to perform, you need know they're doing it correctly. Crafting a sleeve has so many tricks and details. It needs to be designed to give you the maximum outcome down the road. And if you don't have any restriction, I would check with your surgeon's technique and what happened in that procedure.

Chapter 3

Resleeve, Mini Gastric Bypass, Protein & Single Incision

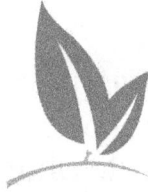

"I prefer the sleeve because it's not that invasive, it doesn't reroute intestines, it doesn't have the malabsorption, malnutrition, malnourishment, vitamin deficiencies that the bypass has or the mini gastric bypass has."

To watch the #AskDrA Show episode that this chapter is based on, follow along at:
www.bit.ly/AskDrA3

How do I know that I am a candidate for a resleeve?

A resleeving, it seems very simple to think, "Okay, I didn't lose enough weight, I want to resleeve myself and get to goal." First, you need to think about what's wrong. Why didn't you get to your goal? Are you eating too many carbs? What are you eating? What was your original bougie size? What was the technique used in your surgery? Who did your surgery? What are outcomes your surgeon is experiencing? What's going on behind the scenes? Don't just think that because you didn't get to your goal or your doctor's goal or even the correct goal that something is wrong.

Think about your starting BMI. Now think, what's your goal BMI? Or maybe, how your surgery was, how it was planned out, what technique was used for your surgery, what are you eating? Take a look at everything before thinking, "All right, I didn't get to goal, I'm going to look into resleeving." Now what? What's the next step? Rethink about resleeving. It's not that simple.

In our case, we suggest patients get a barium sulfate solution test complete with an endoscopy. Then have the results sent to my office. I review it personally. I've turned so many patients down because nothing was wrong with the sleeve. It was the way they were eating. They were eating too many carbs. They were binge eating, trying to push something into that sleeve that's not healthy.

Nothing is wrong with the sleeve, it's what you're deciding to put into the sleeve that creates the problem.

What is your opinion of the mini gastric bypass vs. sleeve for long term results for weight maintenance?

We have really good studies with the mini gastric bypass. We also have really good studies with the gastric sleeve. I personally prefer the sleeve because it's not that invasive, it doesn't reroute intestines, it doesn't have the malabsorption, malnutrition, malnourishment and vitamin deficiencies that the bypass has or the mini gastric bypass has.

The sleeve has many other advantages anatomically speaking. The same entrance of the stomach that you born with stays there. The same exit of the stomach stays there. There's no osteoporosis down the road. It depends on you, what you'd like to have done depending on your BMI and the way you're planning to work with your procedure. If you think you've decided, you're committed, take the step and whatever you decide you're going to do, stick with it. The sleeve has amazing results with high BMI, low BMI patients. It has a lot to do with the patient. So be committed and take the step.

What is your opinion on the single incision?

I don't like it. I've tried it. I've done a few surgeries. But, honestly, I don't think it's a viable solution. That's why we abandoned the procedure right away. Here's why...you don't expand or dissect correctly, you don't get to traction the stomach completely and patients that are non-single incision sleeves get more restriction than the patients with the single incision sleeve. I think a multiple incision surgery has better safety and better outcome for the patient over a single incision sleeve.

Is it true it takes 2 years for your skin to shrink?

Sadly, it's a myth. To think that your skin will shrink back after 2 years is a misconception at best. If you start to exercise after your sleeve, focus on what you're eating, getting your skin well hydrated, that helps, but if you're 2 years down the road and thinking that it's going to actually shrink, it's not. It's going to be loose so you might as well do something or just accept it the way it is but it's a myth that after 2 years, your skin will actually shrink back.

I'm 3 weeks post op, and only supposed to lift 15 pounds. It's a day job with one year olds. If I'm careful should I be fine lifting the kids?

For legal purposes and on the paperwork that we send out to patients, it says that lifting is limited to 5 pounds the first week. After that it's in 5 pound increments every week thereafter.

For practical purposes, it's really easy, just remember, don't lift more than 30 pounds the first 30 days. Need a note for work? We send instructions home for you to follow and can write up restrictions so your employer can adjust your work load.

What is the maximum amount of protein we should consume in a day?

Let's talk about your protein intake. Your maximum amount is actually 2 grams per each kilogram of your ideal weight. It can go from 1 to the maximum 2 grams. That's where it tops off. More than that, it's not recommended. It doesn't help to do extra and less than 1 gram, you're not getting enough protein to regenerate tissues.

Okay, but you're probably thinking darn, I have to do math while trying to lose weight. No worries it's really easy to figure out.

Look, the body cannot absorb more than 30 grams of protein at once, and 50 to 70 grams is the max per day you should consume.

Well if you want to keep it simple spread the protein over the course of the day and it'll work. You'll be fine.

Chapter 4

Raw Veggies, Decaf Coffee and Alcohol Consumption

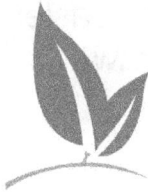

"Raw vegetables and fruits are really good because they don't lose certain nutrients that may get lost if you actually cook them."

To watch the #AskDrA Show episode that this chapter is based on, follow along at:
www.bit.ly/AskDrA4

Is it true that you should not consume raw fruits or vegetables with the sleeve?

Well that's not exactly true. They are indeed really good for you. Raw vegetables and fruits are good because they don't lose certain nutrients that may get lost if you cook them. You need those certain nutrients, certain vitamins, foods that have nutritional value that actually are really good for you. Stay away from them? No way! There is so much benefit from most fruits and vegetables. And it's actually really good for you to consume them raw. Don't stay away from them. Cooking them makes them softer and maybe easier to chew, but they are perfectly safe for you raw.

Why can I consume a large amount of vegetables and fruits with the sleeve compared to protein?

It all has to do with the amount of liquid or fluid the meal or the food has. With fruits and vegetables, you will be able to consume a little bit more. They go down the sleeve easier, because they're more hydrated. They have more water in their content, which actually helps to lubricate and go down the sleeve easier versus protein. When you're talking about protein I'm guessing you're talking more about red meat or chicken or maybe some salmon.

Those are drier. Think about a chicken breast which is really dry. It'll fill you up really quick because it doesn't have moisture in it. Take those dry proteins versus fruits or vegetables that have more fluid. Of course they'll go down easier. That is the reason why you can consume certain amounts of fruits and vegetables more than with certain proteins.

How long do we have to wait before drinking alcohol?

Talking about alcohol, it is very important that you understand that while you're losing weight your metabolism to alcohol is different. Why is this? Well, because you are going through a lot of changes. Your liver is very busy metabolizing all the fatty acids that are being burned in your body because of your new sleeve. Your body is going under a lot of stress while you're losing weight which is good and expected. But when you drink alcohol, what happens is your liver puts a hold on metabolizing that alcohol. Your liver so busy with processing everything else that alcohol is processed last.

Since it puts a hold on the alcohol, your alcohol levels in your blood will start to rise. Incidentally, you will get drunk quicker and the effects lasts longer because the liver is working overtime. So unless you wish to become a very cheap date lay off the alcohol until you reach your goal weight. Once you hit the goal and you stabilize at a certain weight, everything returns back to normal and your free to consume alcohol in moderation.

When can we have decaf coffee?

How does right away sound? Well, almost right away. I can let you know that you can start drinking it right away after surgery once your surgeon gives you the "good to go" with clear liquids. Once you get the go ahead you could start doing decaf. You can even start doing regular coffee once you hit week two or week three after surgery and take off after that. Decaf, since it doesn't have any caffeine, there is no content that irritates the sleeve. But be careful. Make sure it's not too hot, just warm. Don't push the sleeve.

Remember, the first few weeks after surgery the tissue is swollen and it may feel like fire going in. You want to put out the fire, you don't want to put more fire in there, so you want to ease it up. Not too hot, just warm coffee. Decaf you can do right away along with decaffeinated teas which are also allowed. As always check with your doctor. Regarding our practice, you can try it right away.

Chapter 5

Clear Liquids, Complications
& Carbonated Beverages

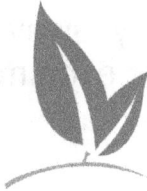

"I always back up my work and offer a guarantee, and make sure that you're going to be just fine, and if anything happens, we can always see you back and we don't charge anything extra."

To watch the #AskDrA Show episode that this chapter is based on, follow along at:
www.bit.ly/AskDrA5

Last November I had gastric sleeve surgery but now I'm drinking 3 cans of diet coke. Is it safe to drink? And, how much can I have?

We always tell patients it's not ideal to be on carbonated beverages. It's just not good. The carbonated gas always irritates the sleeve, so you want to try to avoid drinking them. Is it safe? Yeah, it's safe. Drinking sodas won't cause any issues to the sleeve unless you may have some episodes of gastritis or inflammation. But, of course, we always try to avoid it, so drinking three cans of Diet Coke, I wouldn't recommend it. It's not a good eating habit. You may want to stay away from it, and maybe switch it to some tea or even maybe some water.

I'm at my fifth week and I'm starting to gain weight. I don't know if that is normal or if I should talk to my doctor about it.

Well, it's not normal to have a weight regain at five weeks postop. We may talk about weight regain some years down the road, but not five weeks, I would definitely check with your doctor. We keep up to date with our patients, we follow up with them, so if at five weeks you are experiencing some weight regain, it's definitely a red flag. I would surely consult with your doctor. See what type of technique they have, how the sleeve was crafted, what bougie size they used, because all these factors have an influence on the results you're experiencing.

What happens if you have VSG surgery in Mexico, have complications, but you live in the USA?

Let's talk about complications in Mexico. We get this question a lot. What happens if I get a complication and I go back to the States, then what happens? Well first, I always back up my work by offering a guarantee. Before discharging you we make sure that you're going to be just fine. Now if anything happens, you're welcome to come back and we don't charge anything extra. We take care of you. This is why we always keep you here forty eight hours.

If complications are to occur it's within the first forty eight hours after surgery. Patients may be a little bored. I prefer they're a little bored, and safe here. We check on you to make sure everything is good up to the moment you're discharged. Otherwise, we don't let you go. We make sure you go home safe and sound. And once home, all you have to do is keep on the liquid diet phase and follow along with all the instructions we send with you, and everything will be just fine. Now for what other doctors do, I can't say much about them because not everybody offers the guarantee that we do. And, not everybody has the same connection with their coordinators and doctors that we have with our patients.

How important is it on phase 1 clear liquids to get protein in?

Let's talk about protein and the importance of protein the first week. Since we tell you to do clear liquids, you're limited to certain options when it comes to protein. There are some powders that you can use. On the shopping list we provide you information on what to purchase at the grocery store. Everybody's taste is a little different, so some people tolerate the powders and some people don't. But they can have chicken soup and maybe some whey protein that can be used that first week to get in your liquids. There's also Isopure, or some of the other products that will mix well.

Now, you also have the option of doing the protein shots, the Protein Bullets. They're kind of sweet. Some people don't agree with them, but it's an option. The other option you can do is some broth. Broth has some protein. Then there's flavorless protein powder, you can mix it with juice and some other liquids. You really don't have to focus that much on protein the first week. What I really want you to focus on is hydration. Keeping yourself hydrated is the most important thing on Phase 1. Follow it for seven days. After Phase 1, you jump to Phase 2, which is full liquids where you can incorporate the protein shakes, regular shakes and protein powders.

Chapter 6

Chewing Gum, Counting Carbohydrates & Hair Loss

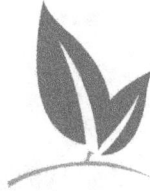

"Keep the carbs under 30 grams and the fat will just melt off!"

To watch the #AskDrA Show episode that this chapter is based on, follow along at: www.bit.ly/AskDrA6

Can I chew gum after having sleeve surgery?

Is it good to chew gum after surgery? Is it safe? It really is safe; it won't put you at risk. But it can be uncomfortable, especially the first few months after surgery. When you chew gum, you're actually swallowing some air, it's coming down in to your newly crafted sleeve (aka your new stomach). That air is actually building up inside your sleeve creating an uncomfortable sensation. That feeling is something I want you to avoid. I don't recommend chewing gum. Switch to hard candy instead, there's no air swallowing involved and no discomfort. I would avoid chewing gum at least the first 3 months after surgery. After 3 months your sleeve will be able to hold that amount of air and you won't have that issue.

Should I be counting carbs... or net carbs?

When you really get into counting carbs, you can actually subtract certain carbs that come from fiber or alcohols from the total carbs you eat in a day. These carbs that come from alcohol or fiber are easily metabolized by your body because they don't spike up your blood sugar. The glycemic index in these types of foods don't have that much impact on your blood sugar and they're very low impact. So, what you want to do is actually subtract the total carbs from these low impact carbs and you get what we call the net carbs. This is a little bit more into counting carbs, and if you've gotten to this point you're doing really good. Of course, I tell patients to try to get to under 30 grams, that will make your fat just melt off. You've got to do this for certain number of days of course, until your metabolism kicks in and that process will start to melt the fat.

Is it normal to lose much hair after surgery?

Not everybody loses hair after surgery. Those that do, you're talking about patients who have experienced a big transformation in weight loss. Patients who lose a lot of weight right away, patients who are smaller in stature but see a transformation in size. People who have a very intense change. Those types of people will see some hair loss. It happens because of stress on the body from hormonal changes and physical changes attributed to rapid weight loss. But don't worry, it's just temporary.

Once the stress goes away and your body is stabilizing at a certain weight, all the hair will regrow back. And honestly, I haven't seen a bald patient so far, so you'll be just fine. My suggestion: take your supplements, add some biotin (if you like) and the hair, skin and nails will look really good. Of course focus on some protein and your multivitamins. You'll be fine, the hair will regrow.

I am 2 months out and have problems eating green things like salads and spinach in particular blows my belly up. Is this normal?

Yes...but it will normalize over time. You see, eating certain greens after surgery, like spinach, kale and lettuce, they're considered fiber. And, anyone who eats a lot of fiber will blow up. Why? It's fiber! Fiber is a like a sponge...it soaks up fluids. Too much fiber in your intestine and it may make you bloated for a few days. I know all about it.

You see, I've been a vegan for the last 7 months and yes, my belly blew up too. It was kind of funny. I blew up like a balloon the first 3 or 4 days. Boy oh boy, was I bloated. But, after about day 4 it went away. My suggestion is keep doing it, and after a few days your body will get used to it. It's good for you, and those types of greens are low carb.

Chapter 7

Eating, Drinking, Supplements & Gallstones

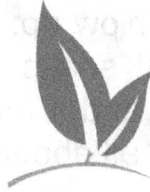

*"Enjoy the weight loss. Eat healthy, and you'll
make the most out of it."*

To watch the #AskDrA Show episode that this
chapter is based on, follow along at:
www.bit.ly/AskDrA7

Is it true that eating then drinking 45 seconds after will stretch your sleeve?

Eating and drinking at the same time is a very common question. Some people think that it'll stretch your sleeve. Some people think that it'll burst your sleeve or damage the sleeve. Nothing will happen to your sleeve people. Nothing will happen to your sleeve.

The reason we tell you to actually stop drinking 30 to 45 minutes before your meal and start drinking again 30 to 45 minutes after your meal is because of 2 things. Number 1, it feels very uncomfortable to have the mixture of solids, fluids at the same time in your sleeve, because it creates a funnel effect. Number 2, is if you avoid the drinking the fluids, you're not flushing food down. It will give you a sensation of fullness much quicker. It's the funnel effect that'll switch the fluids and the solids at the same time. Doesn't feel good at all, so I try to avoid that sensation on you. The other thing is, the swishing or the flushing of solid foods.

Can you take a fat burner before you work out? I'm 3 months out.

If you're thinking of taking some supplements, some fat burners, the answer is yes you can take them but why would you want to take them if you're 3 months out from surgery? You're rocking your sleeve! You're dropping in weight. You're melting that fat off. You're melting those pounds off. Why not just give your sleeve a chance to do its job prior to thinking of fat burners, supplements, and some other stuff? Take your protein. Take your vitamins. Avoid those supplements. You don't need them. You probably were taking them prior to surgery. But, you don't need them right now. You've got your big tool. Explore that tool. Make the most out of it! Stay away from all those supplements.

How much do I need to worry about gallstones after sleeve surgery?

Gallstones after weight loss surgery, vary depending on the procedure. Gastric bypass patients do get the gallstones more than the gastric sleeve. Duodenal switch patients or BPD (below pancreatic diversion) patients, will actually get more than the gastric bypass, and the gastric sleeve more than the lap band. It'll depend on what procedure you had. Let's say you did get your gastric sleeve. How common is it? Well, it depends on if you were meant to have gallstones down the road. Rapid weight loss is known to accelerate gallstones or gall bladder disease.

If you were meant to have it down the road, the procedure and the weight loss will make it more possible that you will get the gall stones sooner. Now, if you get the gallstones, you can get a simple procedure done laparoscopically to remove the gall bladder. Don't worry that much having gastric sleeve and thinking about gallstones down the road. If you do get them, you can get a simple laparoscopic procedure and you're done.

Some physicians will recommend a medication called Actigall. That medication will prevent the gallstones, but once you stop taking the Actigall, if you were meant to have the gallstones, here we go again, those gallstones will appear. I don't recommend it to my patients. Either you were prone to have them, you were meant to have them, you will get them sooner or later. Just don't worry about that. Enjoy the weight loss. Eat healthy, and you'll make the most out of it.

Chapter 8

Acne, Electrolytes & Effects On Your Bones

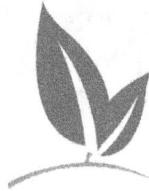

"Take your calcium, put your mind at ease and you'll be just fine."

To watch the #AskDrA Show episode that this chapter is based on, follow along at:
www.bit.ly/AskDrA8

Is it normal to have issue with acne after surgery?

Acne is not directly related to the gastric sleeve, but sometimes the weight loss may cause a hormonal imbalance. That imbalance in particular may cause some acne breakouts. You may want to check with your dermatologist. It's temporary! And, after your body adjusts to the changes all will calm down and everything will be under control. It's very common, mainly with women between the ages of 13 to 45. Then, after your weight loss starts to stall, your body will start to regulate those imbalances and everything will return to normal.

Does this weight loss affect our bones?

This is more related to other bariatric procedures like the gastric bypass. The gastric bypass is directly related to osteoporosis or loss of bone density. It is not directly related to the gastric sleeve, but on people who have that predisposition I would suggest taking calcium. Calcium is recommended for gastric sleeve patients, specifically in women between the ages 18 to 45, to prevent any osteoporosis in the future. Take your calcium, put your mind at ease, and you'll be just fine.

I seem to be getting critical low lab values on my potassium and sodium. What do I do? I'm on a phase 2 diet.

So you're concerned that your low potassium, low sodium is a result of the gastric sleeve surgery? Well, I can assure you that it's not directly related to the gastric sleeve. What I would suspect however, is that its caused by a potassium imbalance or sodium imbalance. And, it's related to medications that you're currently taking. Medications like diuretics for high blood pressure. I would recommend calling your primary health physician. Let them know the problem, adjust the medications or even stop taking them depending on your case. Your doctor will advise and he or she will help you to get those electrolytes balanced and back in check.

Chapter 9

Reflux, Bowel Movements & How Much To Eat

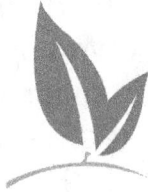

"You have to have a little bit of patience here and wait for nature to do its job."

To watch the #AskDrA Show episode that this chapter is based on, follow along at:
www.bit.ly/AskDrA9

Is it normal to wake up choking after you fall asleep if you have previously eaten with the sleeve?

When you wake up choking after eating, it's reflux. There's no other thing. If you have reflux in the past before the surgery, the surgery may cause some flare ups and may cause an increase of the GERD or the gastroesophageal reflux disease. When you have a sleeve, the worst thing you can do is eat, have dinner, and immediately go to bed. Terrible, terrible! You'll wake up choking.

Why is this? Because before the surgery, you had a big stomach. It could hold quite a bit of food in there. You would lay down and there's still space for the meal or whatever is digesting in there to spread out. With the sleeve, there's no more space. You have dinner, now that food is in a long narrow tube. It's there getting digested and whenever you lay down, you're spilling that digestion gas and guess where it's coming back to? Your throat!

Why? Well, you're laying back flat, gravity will cause it to go to your esophagus and back to your throat. The worst thing you can do is have dinner then go to bed. You'll wake up choking. What you need to do is have early dinner and wait at least two hours before going to bed. Not everybody gets it, but if you do experience GERD, then it's just a slight adjustment to your eating and sleeping habits.

Is it safe to take a laxative daily or every couple days with the sleeve if you have trouble with bowel movements?

Trouble with bowel movements after sleeve? Yes, it's a common thing. First of all, you need to know that after your sleeve, a bowel movement will take a while, sometimes three, four, five days after your sleeve. If you're not bloated, if you're not uncomfortable, you can wait until this naturally happens. Now, if you're bloated, uncomfortable, suffering from constipation, you may take a stool softener or laxative. It's normal, but it's not that frequent. You have to have a little bit of patience here and wait for nature to do its job. Remember that there's nothing in there. There's just liquid! So you need to be a little patient there.

I'm 2 months post op and I can comfortably eat 3/4 to 1 cup of food sometimes, is this normal and is it harmful?

How much should you eat after your sleeve? It actually varies from patient to patient. There's a lot of variables that come into play. Number one is... who is your surgeon? Number two...what technique they used? Number three...what size bougie did they use? Number four...what was your original size of stomach? Number five...how long was it? I could go on and on. All these things or factors come into play to give you the result of your capacity after surgery. Three fourths of a cup or a cup after surgery is not bad. This capacity also varies on patients who are coming from a band, failed lap band to a sleeve. Those patients have even a greater capacity. It's not bad, it just depends on your doctor's technique, bougie used, etc.

Chapter 10

Vitamins, Quantity To Eat & Going Back to The Gym

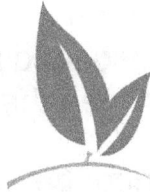

"I don't want you to get overwhelmed with this stuff. Don't let it get to your head."

To watch the #AskDrA Show episode that this chapter is based on, follow along at:
www.bit.ly/AskDrA10

What vitamins are recommended post operation? And in which form? Liquid, gel tab or chewable?

These are questions that unfortunately will vary from doctor to doctor, or practice to practice. Here at Endobariatric we recommend you start one week after your surgery. Why? Because we don't want you bombarding those sleeves with too much medication and vitamins. It's just not good. The sleeve is so swollen that first week that taking too much medication or supplements could have the opposite effect and really upset how you feel. Immediately after sleeve surgery you're going to be taking some medication for your sleeve, an acid blocker, an antibiotic so adding the supplements, vitamins, is not a good idea that first week.

After the first week, once the swelling subsides, you can start with the vitamins. I recommend either liquid, chewable, or gummies. Not regular vitamins. No way. Not yet. Not until you're at least three months out from your gastric sleeve. After those three months, you can take those regular horse pills, no problem. Whatever vitamins you decide that's fine, but those first three months, please don't take big pills. Find them either in a chewable form, gummy or liquid. Do I prefer one or the other? Depends on the brand. I actually like the gummies.

How can I know that the quantity of food I'm eating is adequate for weight loss?

We talked a little bit about this in Chapter 9. First of all, I don't want you to get overwhelmed with this stuff. Don't let it get to your head. As long as you're eating less than half of what you used to eat before surgery, you're good. Adding exercise activities will help increase your metabolic rate. Your sleeve will do the rest.

When do you recommend going back to the gym?

Exercise of any sort should wait at least 10 days after sleeve surgery. Start by walking ten, fifteen minutes. Don't overdo it. You can go back to the gym once you're 30 days after your gastric sleeve surgery. Go easy with the abdominal exercises, crunches, CrossFit and even planking. Wait at least 30 to 40 days before starting to do some of those types of exercises. After 30 days you should be okay to do light weight lifting.

Chapter 11

Vitamin D, Shakes & Allergies

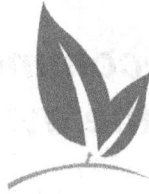

"Don't skip a meal, it's the worst thing you can do with your sleeve."

To watch the #AskDrA Show episode that this chapter is based on, follow along at:
www.bit.ly/AskDrA11

Do gastric sleeve patients live off taking iron, calcium and vitamin D supplements forever?

Taking vitamins, calcium, or even iron for life, is it a must? The answer is no. Some people do require taking some iron supplements and some calcium depending on medical conditions. Women tend to need more calcium and iron. Let me bring you in on a little secret. The first 250 sleeves that I performed back in 2005, 2006, we didn't even give out vitamins because there was no information out there. So if you take a multivitamin now, that's fine, continue to take them. A multivitamin, some calcium, maybe even iron the first year after surgery never hurts. If you're thinking of taking those supplements for life, the answer is no. It's your personal choice.

Is a protein shake enough to kick start my metabolism in the morning?

Do you need to take a protein shake in the morning? The answer is no. Do you have to have something in the morning? The answer is yes. Would that speed up your metabolism, the answer is yes. If nothing agrees with you in the morning and the only thing available because of time, or time consumption or ease of use is a protein shake, then drink a protein shake. That's fine with me. It speeds up metabolism. Don't skip a meal. That's the worst thing you can do with a sleeve. I don't like my patients using protein shakes six months after surgery. I prefer patients having either vegetable or animal protein. Yes, actual protein in their food not from a protein shake.

Is it normal to break out in unexplained hives after surgery?

Allergies after surgery, may be common in some patients who are very allergenic. Examples would be patients who have allergies to certain medications used for pain or allergies to adhesives. The adhesives I'm talking about are in the strips used to cover the incisions. Some patients might be allergic to iodine or even NSAIDS and might break out in hives. If the allergy is severe you might even experience some blisters around your abdomen incisions.

Is it common? No! I'm talking about very specific patients. If it's the case that you break out with some hives what you can do is use some regular Benadryl, or an antihistamine or even topical steroids to help with the allergic reaction. Of course you can always contact us. We'll be on top of things and take care of you along the way. Otherwise if you have surgery with someone else, contact your doctor or your surgical service for their advice.

Chapter 12

Dumping Syndrome, Being Cold & Losing Weight Before Sleeve Surgery

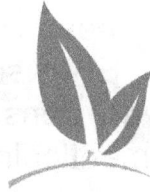

"Once you start losing weight, that fat tissue starts to get thinner and thinner and thinner."

To watch the #AskDrA Show episode that this chapter is based on, follow along at: www.bit.ly/AskDrA12

What is Dumping Syndrome?

Okay, let's talk about Dumping Syndrome. It's something very commonly seen in gastric bypass patients, but it's not that common with gastric sleeve patients. You're talking about a very small minority of the patients that may have what we call a Dumping Syndrome. Five to seven percent of patients may experience Dumping Syndrome with the gastric sleeve. The name alone sounds awful doesn't it? So, let me explain what Dumping Syndrome is all about.

When we talk about syndrome, it's a combination of symptoms a patient may have. Symptoms like tachycardia, rapid heart rate, palpitations, sweatiness, dizziness. Even some nausea or even vomiting after eating very dense food. Talking about dense food, we're mentioning about very high concentrated sugars, shakes, or very high fiber foods that may enter your GI tract. What happens is very high concentrations of food go into your sleeve and rapidly enter the first portion of your intestine and will trigger this syndrome.

Why didn't you have it before surgery? The reason is very simple, because you did have a big pouch of stomach. And, it was able to hold food for longer periods of time. Then once that food was digested and diluted with saliva it passed into your intestine.

Not anymore. With the sleeve, you have a very small stomach, that will actually hold food for a while and then pass it along into your intestine. It's this rapid passing of food that triggers this syndrome. Don't get overwhelmed with this. Remember, a very small minority of the patients will develop this syndrome. Easily treated by avoiding eating copious amounts of foods with high concentrations of sweets or sugars.

Is it normal to be cold a lot since weight loss surgery?

The simple answer...yes!

The more complicated answer has to do with a layer of fatty tissue underneath your skin. That layer of fat tissue may be big or small or in between. Everybody has it no matter how thin you are. That fat tissue, sometimes referred to as a "fat pad" actually serves as a temperature barrier. Once you start losing weight, that fat tissue starts to get thinner and thinner and thinner. You still have it, but it's now in a thinner layer.

Think of it this way...instead of having a very big jacket to ward against the weather, now you have a very thin layered jacket which allows the cold sensation in. Your body was adjusted to a certain set point, but now that the fat tissue is gone your body is perceiving the outer temperature in a very new way.

I need to lose 50 pounds before surgery, I already changed my eating habits, I've gained weight. What should I do now?

Let's talk about the pre-op diet and why you have to lose some weight before surgery. It's not because I want to give you a hard time or your surgeon wants to give you a hard time. It's because we want to give you the best outcome possible. If you don't lose weight, if don't adhere to the liquid diet, if you don't follow the instructions, you will not lose what we call the visceral fat. Visceral fat is the fat around the organs. But most importantly it's about your liver size at the time of surgery. If you don't lose the weight, you will not shrink your liver and surgery in some cases, won't be possible. You need to be very compliant with your surgeon's rules and what he or she needs you to lose before the surgery.

Chapter 13

Acid Blockers, Age Range & Sore Muscles

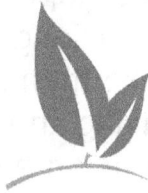

"I pick every patient in particular, and analyze their health history to make sure he or she is a good candidate for the gastric sleeve."

To watch the #AskDrA Show episode that this chapter is based on, follow along at:
www.bit.ly/AskDrA13

I've read that long term use of PPI's can cause bone loss. Is this something we should be concerned about?

Some acid blockers such as PPIs (proton pump inhibitors), omeprazole, pantoprazole and others are known to cause some lowering of calcium in blood. Which could lead to osteoporosis down the road. It's a mixed feeling. We have some good medical articles that support using them. And, we've got good medical articles that say that it's not true. The question is, what happens if you take acid blockers like PPIs for a long period of time? The thing is, if you don't take them, the risk of not taking them is more than taking them. You need to take them. You can bring it down a notch, you don't have to take the PPIs forever. You can take H2 blockers like ranitidine, which is Zantac in the US. If that works for you, stick to it. Zantac doesn't have those side effects. If it brings the acid down, you can keep on using it.

What is the least age for a person to have the sleeve surgery?

Our youngest patient was twelve years old at the time of surgery. Our oldest patient was seventy four. These were very particular cases. We try to keep the guidelines between eighteen to sixty five. We analyze the health history of every patient and make sure he or she is a good candidate for the gastric sleeve. Their overall health is very important and if something doesn't look right or may pose a risk we don't operate. Remember the sleeve is an elective surgery. If the patient is younger or older than the guidelines we evaluate to make sure everything is perfect.

I have extremely sore muscles and I have to work. What can I take to ease the pain?

Okay, so you have some muscle soreness or a headache and you want to know what you can use to feel better? If you were thinking about taking Advil, I would say...the answer is no. You see, Advil is part of the NSAID family. Not recommended! Maybe you remember in a prior chapter that we talked about this before. We try to avoid those medications. Your best option is always Tylenol, either liquid, gel cap or regular tablet. You can take regular tablets after three months remember? Liquid gel caps are good. Tylenol is always the best option.

Chapter 14

Heartburn, Dizziness & Hiatal Hernia

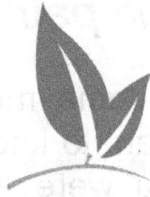

"Because your body is changing, becoming smaller, so is your cardiovascular system, your heart, your lungs, the amount of blood, the amount of fluid in your body, all these systems have to adjust to the new you."

To watch the #AskDrA Show episode that this chapter is based on, follow along at:
www.bit.ly/AskDrA14

I have developed almost constant heartburn. I took Omeprazole and the heartburn is a little bit better. Will I need to take medication forever?

Having heartburn is common, especially with patients who had heartburn before surgery. If you have heartburn before surgery, it will probably continue for a while after. Now, normally, the acid production of the stomach increases after the sleeve, so you will have to take some antacids for a while. Sometimes, it's a few days. Sometimes, a few months. Sometimes, it may be a couple of years. Then, this acid production normally lowers as the years go by. Is it mandatory to take the acid blockers forever? The answer is no. Normally, it's a few weeks to a few months.

I have occasional dizzy spells due to low blood pressure. Causes and remedies?

Being dizzy after surgery is actually really common. This is because your body is adjusting to the new you. Why? Because your body is changing, becoming smaller, so your cardiovascular system, your heart, your lungs, the amount of blood, the amount of fluid in your body, all these systems have to adjust to the new you. Once it adjusts, your body still keeps changing and you may continue having these dizzy spells. They're normal. I would recommend avoiding really rapid movements like tying your shoelaces and then standing up really quick. Rapid movements will trigger those dizzy spells. Not everybody gets them, but if you do, try to avoid those rapid movements. They will go away once your body adjusts and once you're stabilized and you're not losing any more weight.

Are you still able to have VSG if you have a hernia?

Are you a candidate if you have a hiatal hernia? The answer is yes. Actually, most of our patients don't even know they have a hiatal hernia. Thirty to forty percent of patients that go in for a gastric sleeve have no idea they have a hiatal hernia. They have some indigestion, maybe some heartburn. During surgery, we go in and we discover it. What do we do? We fix it of course! And, in our case, we don't charge extra, so our patients get a 2 for 1 bundle. The idea is to fix the hiatal hernia since we're already there. We fix it and we do the sleeve in one step. So the answer is yes, if you do have a hiatal hernia you can still have the VSG procedure. The heartburn gets taken care of, and you get your gastric sleeve.

Chapter 15

Thyroid, Bruising, Hot Tubs & Straws

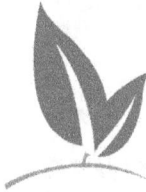

"Let the incisions heal naturally."

To watch the #AskDrA Show episode that this chapter is based on, follow along at:
www.bit.ly/AskDrA15

What do you recommend our TSH at?

I get questions regularly of people asking me what is a good level of TSH, that's the thyroid hormone. All right, here goes. It is important for you to understand that the sleeve is very independent from your thyroid. Your thyroid levels will be different then someone else. They vary from person to person. If you have thyroid issues before surgery, please follow up with your endocrinologist, because he or she will be the one to ask, "What are my thyroid levels, what should they be, and what to do about them?" Please separate your sleeve from your thyroid; totally independent.

I have a lot of bruises, is this normal?

Bruising after surgery, fairly common, but I would suggest you get some blood work done. Number one, check your blood work. Make sure there's no other thing causing the bruising. From a standpoint of sleeve surgery, bruising is not that common. I would check your blood work. Check with your PCP. Make sure your blood levels, your platelet levels, your iron levels and your hemoglobin are all good. Stuff that your PCP will take care of and coach you.

I wouldn't worry that much regarding your sleeve. I would check first any other issue that may be related to the bruises.

When can I go into a hot tub?

The answer to submerging underwater after surgery varies from practice to practice. At Endobariatric, we recommend our patients not to submerge underwater like a bathtub, swimming pool or hot tub in the first 15 days. Let the incisions heal naturally. After 15 days, after those incisions are healed, you can submerge underwater. Before 15 days, the last thing you want to worry about is a skin infection. Try to avoid submerging underwater.

Are we never going to be able to use a straw?

Straws are normally not recommended. But, I tell my patients small straws, like the ones used with the small juices, or the Hi-C juices, those you can use right away. I wouldn't recommend using regular straws right after surgery because when you suck on the straw, a column of air first comes in through your mouth, and you end up swallowing that air. That air will end up in your sleeve and may cause discomfort the first 3 months after surgery. After 3 months, your sleeve will be able to handle regular straws. I would avoid using straws initially.

Chapter 16

Low Energy, OTC Medications
& The Flu Vaccine

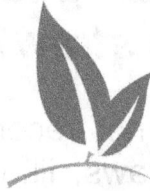

*"Make sure you're resting at least eight hours
during the evening and taking your supplements."*

To watch the #AskDrA Show episode that this
chapter is based on, follow along at:
www.bit.ly/AskDrA16

I'm 6 days post operation and I have no energy. Is this normal?

Yes. I would recommend you get some rest and make sure you're not overdoing it. Make sure you're resting at least eight hours during the evening and taking your supplements. The other thing is, if you are not consuming enough calories, you may hit a wall with low energy. That is why the first few weeks after surgery we do recommend you include some carb intake in your diet. You need those carbs to keep a good level of energy. Right after surgery, clear liquids. We do encourage patients to drink regular juice with sugar, because well when you go the other way with light or sugar-free, you may hit the low energy wall that I'm talking about. Make sure your carb consumption is good, make sure you are resting well and that you are not overdoing it.

Can we take any kind of cold/allergy medications?

The answer is no. Now if you ask, "Can I take common over the counter medication for flu?" The answer is yes. Just make sure you're not taking any anti-inflammatories that may harm your sleeve. You can take Benadryl, you can take antihistamines, you can even take stuff for runny nose. It won't harm your sleeve. Not sure what can you should take? The best thing is to run it by me or your surgeon. My patients have my direct email and you can always touch base with me. If you're not my patient, I would recommend to touch base with your PCP or your surgeon. Make sure you're on the safe side.

Should we have our flu vaccine before or after our surgery?

If you're thinking about the flu shot, then I would suggest getting your shot done at least two weeks prior to your surgery. The vaccine typically takes about two weeks to work through and strengthen your immune system. Now, if decide to wait until after surgery to get the shot then please wait at least two to three weeks. Your body needs time to recover from surgery. Once you're recovered and you're doing well and maintaining a good level of energy then get your shot.

My recommendation: get it done before surgery.

Chapter 17

Slimy Saliva, Gastric Emptying & Nexium Antacid

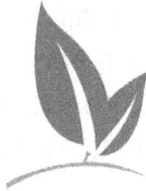

"Remember the sleeve is crafted for solids and not for liquids."

To watch the #AskDrA Show episode that this chapter is based on, follow along at:
www.bit.ly/AskDrA17

I'm 1-month post op. Is it normal to wake up with dry mouth and sticky saliva?

All those who have had a sleeve know about the slimy saliva. It's a thick saliva that's common in patients with very tight sleeves, or in patients whose sleeve has actually gotten swollen. Normally you see it in the mornings. Why? The simple reason is, you've been asleep throughout the whole night and that saliva has a chance to build up. When you wake up you may experience the slimy saliva...hey, it's normal! Nothing weird. No alien is building inside of you! It's totally expected on patients with a sleeve. If you don't like all that saliva, here's what you can do...a round or two of antacids for 2 or 3 weeks and that will take care of it. If you do the rounds of antacids and they don't go away, contact your doctor.

How much time does it take for the stomach to empty fluids?

This is more like a physiological question. What happens right away if you drink water? What happens to the water? Does it sit in your stomach, does it empty right away, does it sit there for long periods of time. So here's the simple answer...the liquid goes right through the sleeve, it doesn't sit there long enough. It empties quite rapidly then goes into your intestine.

Now, some people, the first or the second week after their surgery, say "I'm drinking water, I don't feel any restriction, I don't feel full with water." Here's what's happening...those liquids are most likely phase 1 clear liquids. Maybe that patient's sleeve got a little too swollen and there isn't much space. When you pour water in, it actually pours right out into the intestine, it doesn't sit there. Remember that the sleeve is crafted for solids and not for liquids.

Should I worry if I take 2 pills daily of Nexium?

No, Nexium will not cause any issues regarding your sleeve. Nexium is actually one of the best medications or antacids, it's a PPI medication. These medications are really good to protect your stomach. They help protect the swollen tissue after your sleeve surgery. Patients do really well with the Nexium; twenty milligrams in the morning then twenty milligrams in the evening that's forty milligrams throughout the day. If you're actually splitting it 20 and 20, that's fine. You may actually find the Nexium which is 40 milligrams, one pill, you can take that once a day and you're good too.

Chapter 18

Gas, Elevated Liver Enzymes & Converting A Gastric Bypass

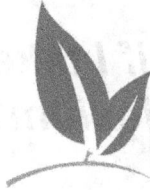

"Everybody wants a sleeve, everybody does good with a sleeve."

To watch the #AskDrA Show episode that this chapter is based on, follow along at:
www.bit.ly/AskDrA18

I'm 7 months out and have gas all the time. Why is this happening?

You should understand there are three types of "gas". There is the gas you experience in your stomach that's is easily treated and the gas that we use to blow up the abdomen to create that space so we can work in and then there is colonic gas.

Let's talk about the second one first. That gas gets absorbed into your body over the next six to twelve hours. In our case, we use a special device that eliminates practically all the gas. Maybe you're left with one or two percent with the gas there, that gets absorbed within a few hours after surgery. That gas after twelve, twenty-four hours, no longer exists.

Now onto the first type of gas. The stomach gas. This one is the most uncomfortable one, and it's the type of gas that builds up in your sleeve. Since the sleeve is so tight, it's virtually a closed space. It's so swollen that nothing fits in there, but some gas may build up, from swallowing air. That gas that you swallow, it builds up in your stomach, and gets very uncomfortable. You can't burp the gas because it's stuck in there. It's actually trapped between the inflammations of your sleeve.

Now, let's talk about colonic gas, that's intestinal gas. I see some people bring their own Gas-X strips and some other medications, and that's more for intestinal gas, which normally sleeve patients don't have. In this case, the patient is seven months out and is having gas. I would recommend they take a round of antacids to get that sleeve unswollen and that should take care of it. If it doesn't, they should contact their surgeon, contact their surgical group to determine what's going on. Normally the antacids take care of it. I hope that clears everything up regarding all the gas.

I have slightly high bilirubin levels, is this normal?

We normally don't see elevated bilirubin levels in patients. I say normally because it's just a low occurrence. When it does show up its auto-limiting and resolves by itself in a manner of weeks. It can also happen when a patient had a bleeder during surgery, or a blood clot, there's a little blood in the abdomen that's getting absorbed, that may elevate liver enzymes, especially the bilirubin levels.

That's what we normally see in the vast minority of the patients. It's not that common. Yes, certain patients that do go into weight loss surgery, and do go under the knife, may get a temporary rise of their liver enzymes that's normal. We monitor those elevated liver enzymes over the next few weeks, and usually they return to normal. I would contact your doctor and schedule a follow up.

Can I have a sleeve after RNY?

This happens to be a very common question. I get it on the boards, in my email, and even in conversation and it starts out like this... "I had a gastric bypass done years ago. Can I convert that to a sleeve?" The sleeve is the big hot topic nowadays. Everybody wants one! The answer to the question may surprise you, "In theory, yes you can, but in practice no." It's very difficult and it's practically useless to convert a very complex surgery, which is the gastric bypass, to a much simpler procedure, which is the gastric sleeve.

It would involve reattaching the upper part of your stomach to the regular big stomach, plus, then detaching your intestine which is connecting to the upper part of your stomach back to your regular intestine, and then, perform a sleeve. It just doesn't make sense. The sleeve is practically just a vertical cut, cut the rest out and leave the banana shaped stomach. In theory, yes, it can be done, in practice it's not practical. You will not get much benefit out of it, so why perform it.

Chapter 19

C-pap Machine, High Protein/Low Carb Diet & Vitamins/Supplements

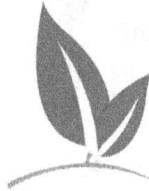

"I would focus on a greener vegetable fruit diet and drop all the junk food."

To watch the #AskDrA Show episode that this chapter is based on, follow along at:
www.bit.ly/AskDrA19

When can we use a C-pap without the fear of swallowing air and blowing out stitches?

This is more a myth than anything else. There are no scientific studies, there is really nothing out there regarding using a C-PAP machine after gastric sleeve surgery. The fear that a CPAP machine designed for people with sleep apnea will pump too much air into your recently done sleeve and blow it up is misplaced at best. It just doesn't happen.

We do surgeries on a lot of people who have sleep apnea, on a lot of people who use a CPAP machine, or the BPAP machine. Let me tell you a little bit about these machines. These machines are automatic. They are so automatic that they sense the breathing cycle of the patient. They will not push more or less air in. They follow the breathing pattern of the patient, so that air goes directly to the lungs while you're breathing while you're asleep. There is no way that this air will go directly to your sleeve or it will pump a lot of air in to blow it up.

It's just a myth...nothing to fear. If you use a CPAP machine, it's because you need it, so use it.

Is low carb/high protein the only diet recommended after sleeve surgery or are there other diets to follow once you've reached goal?

We're jumping into touchy subjects now. It's seems lately everyone wants to know... "What diet do you recommend after the sleeve?" Well, I push my patients to do a low carb diet high in protein. Why? Well, if I tell them, "Alright, forget about the protein. Just focus on eating healthy. Cut the junk food out. Focus on a lot of leafy products. Focus on a lot of vegetables. Focus on a lot of fruits." The vast majority of my patients will not follow that diet.

So, the easiest way I've come up with that patients do well with, is lowering their carb consumption and keeping them on a good amount of protein per day. Now, a good amount of protein per day does not mean I want you drinking shakes or downing supplements all day long. Just focus on just healthy food. After three or four months, drop the shakes, drop the supplements. You don't need them because the protein will come from what you eat. You will not have a deficiency of protein. Believe me!

Now, I would recommend that your diet focus on greener vegetables and fruit and drop all the junk food. Make wise decisions.

Do you recommend taking vitamins and supplements all at once or split them up throughout the day?

This question was posted by a non-patient on our Facebook page. How do I know they weren't a patient? Well, I spend a great deal of time educating my patients, they know when they should and shouldn't take their vitamins and supplements. But if you're reading this and you're not a patient here's my answer...taking vitamins and supplements all at once is a big no no. After your sleeve has healed maybe you can do this down the road. But, the first six months, space them throughout the day. Yep, space out your multivitamin, space out your calcium, space out your iron, etc. Don't take everything together. You have a brand new stomach, a tiny stomach, one that needs to be taken care of. I don't want you stacking up the medications in that sleeve. Too much medications and vitamins will get it irritated or upset. Space them out in thirty to forty-five minute increments in the morning and evening depending on how many you need to take.

Chapter 20

Chemotherapy, Night Sweats & Hormone Replacement Therapy

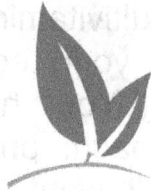

"Make sure everything you're putting in your sleeve is keeping it nice and calm."

To watch the #AskDrA Show episode that this chapter is based on, follow along at:
www.bit.ly/AskDrA20

Chemo is causing havoc on my sleeve. I have gastritis and its tough. Any tips with breast cancer and the sleeve?

I'm really sorry to hear about the diagnosis of breast cancer. I've had quite a few patients that had to battle Lymphoma, breast cancer, prostate cancer, renal cancer, etc., years after getting sleeve surgery. Yes, chemotherapy with or without the sleeve is very aggressive on the body. It can cause gastritis. In this case it is mandatory that antacids or PPI's are constantly used day and night. Yes, morning and evening.

In previous chapters we talked about Nexium and omeprazole. You can use these medications. These products will help protect your sleeve. Number one is take your antacid. Make sure everything you're putting in your sleeve is keeping it nice and as calm as possible. If you are dealing with a lot of nausea, make sure your taking your anti-nausea medication like Zofran or Desitron. Those medications help eliminate or block the nausea, which helps prevent the vomiting. So keeping the sleeve free from irritation is key.

My best advice is to keep your doctor in the loop.

Is it normal to sweat so much at night while sleeping?

The answer is no, it's not normal. There are several reasons for sweating at night. Sometimes it's a hormonal imbalance. Sometimes it can be as simple as having too much coffee throughout the day. Maybe you picked up a new habit. Or you consumed an energy drink and that's what's causing the night sweats. You need to analyze what's going on.

Can the sleeve cause night sweats? No. My recommendation: schedule with your primary care physician and review your everyday habits and see if you can pinpoint what might be causing the night sweats. If it's a hormonal imbalance your doctor will advise. If it's an everyday substance than you know to avoid it.

I'm on hormonal injections and I'm worried if I will be able to continue after my sleeve or will have to stop it. Any recommendations?

Hormone injections or hormonal therapy or replacement therapy, do you need to interrupt it because of the surgery? No. Do you need to wait after your sleeve? No. Do you need to do anything special because of your sleeve? No. Do you need to do anything because you're recovering from your sleeve? The answer is no. The best advice is work with your doctor. Let your surgeon know about this. Let your endocrinologist know about this or your primary health physician know about this and continue taking your medications unless stated by your doctor.

Chapter 21

Weight Stalls, IBS & Plastic Surgery

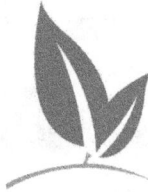

*"Your activity level is very important, so you need
to pick it up."*

To watch the #AskDrA Show episode that this
chapter is based on, follow along at:
www.bit.ly/AskDrA21

Any recommendation to lose my last 10 pounds to reach my goal?

So you want to talk about the weight stalls and losing those few last pounds? Well, they may be a little more difficult but remember that it's always easier to lose the large majority of the pounds you have but those last few pounds can be a little tricky.

The solution is... you need to watch out for the amount of carb intake that you're consuming. You need to avoid the junk food and the snacking. You also need to increase your exercise activity. That activity level is very important, so you need to pick it up. Those two solutions, watching what you're eating and increasing your activity level will give you the solution to losing those few pounds and the weight stalls.

Remember that the weight stalls are healthy and are needed. The stalls help your body recover from the weight loss. They help balance your system out. So some weight stalls throughout your journey are normal. Now, if you have those weight stalls after a year and half, two years and you've hit a plateau, and you want to kick start your weight loss again, you need to decrease your snacking and increase your exercises.

How does the IBS effect the sleeve?

The truth is, IBS (irritable bowel syndrome) has nothing to do with the gastric sleeve. It's totally independent. If you do have IBS with a sleeve, it will continue. It has no relationship whatsoever. It's those things that may get a little bit better because you're eating a bit less, but it will continue.

Will we need plastic surgery after the gastric sleeve?

If you're considering plastic surgery after the gastric sleeve, you need to wait at least 12 months and sometimes probably a little longer to have it performed. Depending on how much weight you need to lose you might even have to wait 18 months. If you are at the 18-month mark and you're still losing weight, then wait until a little longer. Not all my sleeve patients opt for plastic surgery.

It depends on your result at the end of the line. Sometimes my patients don't need anything, no extra skin left over, no nothing, so don't worry about that. Focus on your weight loss and enjoy the journey.

Chapter 22

Menstrual Cycles, Staying Hydrated & Radiation

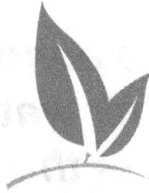

"The key to staying hydrated, especially those first few months, sip & wait, sip & wait."

To watch the #AskDrA Show episode that this
chapter is based on, follow along at:
www.bit.ly/AskDrA21

Is it normal to have my period again if I just had it one week ago before my surgery?

Yes, very common to have menstrual cycle changes after surgery. Why is this? Two main mechanisms. One is stress. You just had surgery. Stress changes hormones, causes hormonal imbalances and it's causing you to either have your period earlier a little after. The other thing is, once you start losing weight, drastic weight loss causes also an imbalance.

Since my sleeve a month ago, every time I try to drink water, it gives me nausea. Why is this happening?

You've got to keep two things in mind, initially, you're at the top peak of restriction. Water may not agree with you for the first two or three months. You may want to add a little extra packet of iced tea or flavored Crystal Light, something that changes the texture of the water so it'll go down nicely. The other thing is, after a few months water will agree with you. It's your own regular stomach as before surgery, so don't worry about that.

The key to staying hydrated, especially those first few months, sip and wait, sip and wait. Always quantify. It's very important. If you don't quantify, you don't know how much water your taking in, so you need to keep up a record, a diary of how much water intake you are having.

I just started chemo and radiation this week. Will this damage my sleeve?

The answer is no. The best advice is, tell your oncologist about your sleeve so he or she can actually keep it well. I would also recommend some antacids or PPI medication to keep your sleeve in good shape while they're giving you a big amount of radiation or chemotherapy treatment.

Chapter 23

Hiccups, Outdoor Activities & Vitamin Patches

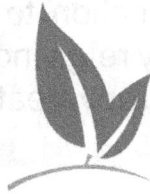

"Have fun, enjoy your sleeve, enjoy your outdoor activities now that you're losing weight."

To watch the #AskDrA Show episode that this chapter is based on, follow along at:
www.bit.ly/AskDrA23

What is the cause of hiccups? Too much air, eating too fast or eating too much?

There's different types of hiccups. One that you get right after surgery and one that you get down the road. They're very different. The one that you get right after surgery, that is related to the swollen tissue and the phrenic nerve. The phrenic nerve is a nerve very close to the esophagus and sleeve. When the sleeve gets swollen right after surgery it pinches the phrenic nerve, which in turn irritates the nerve and causes your esophagus to hiccup.

There is a very small percentage of patients that may get hiccups as a sign that they're full. Some people tell us, "You know what, when I have that last bite, and I get the hiccups, it's like a trigger and it lets me know that's when I'm full." That's actually a good thing to have, if you get the hiccups it's a sign you're full.

Did you know after surgery men get hiccups much more than women do? Yep. it's true.

Is it okay to ride my four-wheeler? I'm almost 4 weeks post op.

Let's talk a little bit about outdoor activities. After four weeks you can pretty much ride a bicycle, you can ride a four-wheeler, you can go horseback riding, pretty much anything. You may be a little extra sore on that left side, that's where the biggest incision was for your sleeve surgery. It will be a little extra sore there. Other than that, feel free to do all that exciting stuff, you won't damage anything inside. What's done is done, what's healed is healed, so jump on the horse, jump on the four-wheeler, jump on the bike. Have fun, enjoy your sleeve, enjoy your outdoor activities now that you're losing weight.

What is your opinion about vitamin patches?

Depends on your needs, but for me they're a little uncomfortable to be placing a patch on my skin every day. For me it's much simpler to grab some gummy vitamins and toss them in my mouth. I think it's easier just to take your multivitamin and you're done. The patches are a good idea, but they may come loose if you take a shower, when you're swimming, relaxing in the bathtub, all that wet stuff.

Those are the inconvenient things that I see with a vitamin patch. Other than that, they're proven to absorb the vitamins as you would do taking them.

They do work. It's lifestyle choice.

Chapter 24

Incision Pain, Juicing, Energy Drinks & Supplements

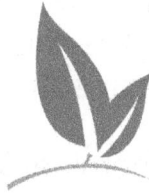

"Your food is your best medication!"

To watch the #AskDrA Show episode that this chapter is based on, follow along at:
www.bit.ly/AskDrA24

I'm a week and a half out from surgery, I get some pain in the area of the stomach and often near the stitches. But am now wondering, if I popped a stitch.

Let's talk about incision pain. You may experience some incision pain usually stemming from the left side close to your midline, that one is the biggest incision. Yes, it will be sore. It may be a little extra tender right there, especially when you do a lot of abdominal exercises, core abdominal muscle crunching, ab work, getting out of bed, bending over, especially the first few weeks after surgery. You may also experience this discomfort down the road if you do very extraneous exercise.

Let's say you do abdominal crunches or you did something different that you put those muscles to work, and maybe looks sore on that left side. It's normal because that's the side where we pull that big chunk of stomach out during the surgery. That is the only incision that has a big stitch through the abdominal wall, and that is what is uncomfortable after your surgery.

That little extra soreness reminds you to take it easy and not over exert yourself which could lead to having a hernia down the road. So take it easy, let it heal and the pain will go away.

How long after surgery can we begin juicing in moderation?

You can start juicing right away after surgery, but try to make those juices clear. Thin them out. Juices are really good. They have a good amount of fructose (natural fruit sugar) which gives you a lot of energy. They have a lot of vitamins and minerals, and they're really good for you.

Remember to thin it out and keep it clear for Phase 1 and a little thicker more color under Phase 2.

After 1-year post op can I drink energy drinks and take supplements?

I actually advise my patients to stop all consumption of those energy drinks. I don't like them. I don't like them at all. I don't like them a few weeks out. I don't like them a year out. I wouldn't suggest drinking the energy drinks. Plus, some of the energy drinks are carbonated, which add unnecessary gas to your sleeve. I don't like the gassy stuff, so I would avoid them. Now supplements, it really depends, because the question is, "Can I drink the energy drinks and take supplements?" Supplements, if you're talking about protein shakes, I don't like them. People, I like my patients to use some supplements the first few weeks after surgery, but after you start eating, your food is your best medication. It's your best supplement. It's your regular food. Drop the protein shakes. Drop the protein bars. Start doing regular food and drop the energy drinks. You don't need them.

Chapter 25

E-cigarettes, Binders
& Losing Sizes But Not Pounds

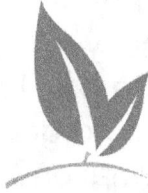

"Patience...this is something that's expected while you're losing weight."

To watch the #AskDrA Show episode that this chapter is based on, follow along at:
www.bit.ly/AskDrA25

Is it okay to use e-cigarettes after surgery?

Do I recommend e-cigarettes? Of course you're asking a doctor. I would say no. To use an e-cigarette versus a regular cigarette, I would prefer the e-cigarette. Remember you're taking this step to change your complete lifestyle. Why not just drop it completely? I know that nicotine is sometimes needed. I know some people struggle with nicotine. Why not just make the complete switch? Now, if you're my patient I'm going to ask you to be off the smoking before and off the smoking after. A few weeks before, a few weeks after. While you're healing inside. It's very important. Why not just continue doing that so you'll know that you really don't need it? It's just a bad habit. It's easy to grab, right? It's also easy not to grab. Why not just make the complete transformation? Coming back to the question. Do I recommend them? Of course not. Do I recommend them verses regular cigarettes? Yeah. Less toxins in there. Less toxins that goes into your body.

Would you recommend to use shape-wear after surgery?

Do you need the shape wear? The answer is no. Do I like them? The answer is still no. Let me explain. With the shape wear (or body shapers or binders), at least the first 6 weeks you will have the incisions healing, and the shape wear holds a lot of humidity and heat in. If you live in a place where already very hot, or the humidity is very high, the incisions will get a little moist. The last thing you want to worry about is a skin infection. And an infection getting into those incisions is the last thing you want to worry about. The skin is very simple and it heals naturally and sometimes very rapidly. But tiny incisions, you have to worry about them.

Don't use shape wear unless you're at least some 6 weeks out, and you need to use them for a certain reason. Otherwise, forget about them.

Why is it possible to drop in inches and not in pounds?

Hey Doc, "I'm losing some sizes, but the scale doesn't move." My reply is always the same, "That's totally normal." Remember some weight stalls are normal, they're needed while your body is adjusting to losing the sizes. You need to have some patience. Remember, just keep doing what you're doing. Keep doing some exercises, don't eat junk food, and sooner or later the inches will stop and the pounds will drop off and the scale will move. Have patience! It's totally normal. This is something that's expected while you're losing weight.

Chapter 26

Stomach Gurgles, Ibuprofen & Resetting Your Sleeve's Restriction

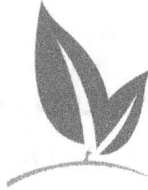

"Don't freak out just watch what you're eating."

To watch the #AskDrA Show episode that this chapter is based on, follow along at:
www.bit.ly/AskDrA26

I'm 2 years out, I frequently and randomly have stomach gurgles just like I did when I was first sleeved. Why?

When your sleeve was initially done it gurgled. We talked about this is in the very first chapter. Now, you're two years out and all of a sudden it's gurgling again. What is going on? It's quite simple. It all has to do with swollen tissue. Right after the surgery, your sleeve is very swollen. There isn't enough space for water, saliva or anything to go down. When it finally makes its way down it will produce this gurgling noise.

Remember? Do you also remember the funnel analogy we talked about? If you have a very narrow funnel, and you're pouring some liquid in quickly, it will gurgle. The reason is that it's a lot of liquid in a very narrow space, and it will produce these gurgling noises.

What can you do to actually get it going or even eliminate these sound? It's quite simple. You need to take an acid blocker for at least three or four weeks. Morning and evening, religiously. It will make a difference, it will get that swollen tissue down, it will open the space, and of course the saliva, the liquids, will be free to flow into your sleeve. The gurgling will go away. In other words, what you're going to be doing is actually making that funnel much larger, and of course you won't be able to gurgle now. I hope that makes sense.

Are we allowed to have ibuprofen (Advil)? If not, why?

Ibuprofen is an over the counter medication used for pain; muscle aches, headaches, menstrual cramps, etc. We don't recommend it for sleeve patients because it belongs to a family of medications called NSAIDS. NSAIDS, which stand for Non-Steroidal Anti-Inflammatory Drugs. These drugs, even without a sleeve, are very aggressive to the inner layer, called the mucosa. It's very easy for patients who are used to taking it for long periods of time to bleed from the stomach. Now with the sleeve, you have a tiny stomach, you need to be careful, much more than before the surgery.

I wouldn't recommend it, unless you just have to take it, let's say you take it once a month for menstrual cramps. If you take them for one of two days, that's fine. You won't have an issue there. If you take ibuprofen every single day, believe me, it will put a hole in your stomach. It will produce an ulcer that may bleed and may get you in trouble. Remember, this is not because of the sleeve, this is because that's what NSAIDS do, right? With or without a sleeve, try to avoid these medications. The best medication for pain or headaches is Tylenol. Tylenol is not a member of the NSAID family and you can take it safely without worrying about your sleeve.

Can the sleeve be reset to go back to feeling original restriction?

Can you reset your sleeve? No. Can you reset to original restriction point? No. Let me tell you why. You're probably aren't comparing yourself to the initial phase, or the postop period where the restriction is at its highest point. What you need to do here is to compare yourself not to those points, but to what you're eating right now. If you're a year out, maybe two years out, compare yourself to what you were eating before surgery. Before you had your sleeve.

If you're comparing yourself to before your sleeve and you're eating about 3 maybe 4 or 5 (on a scale from one to ten) but before surgery you were at a 10 then you're doing fine. Yep, under a five, you're great. That's perfect. That's where you want to be. Of course, right after surgery, you were probably at a one, maybe a two. Now you're eating about a five and you notice that big change, and you're like, "Damn, all right. Now I need to put a lot more effort to this. I don't want to regain some weight." Remember, compare yourself to before the surgery, not right after the surgery.

Let me tell you why the difference. Right after the surgery you've got all that swollen tissue. You've got everything crammed up. There's not much space in there. Remember, you're barely able to sip some water. There's no way you can actually reset that sleeve to that initial post op point, because there's no way to activate all that swollen tissue to create that virtual space just right after surgery.

Please don't freak out. You just need to watch what you eat.

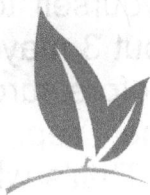

Glossary of Terms

Acid Reflux – is a chronic condition caused by stomach acid coming up into the esophagus

Acne – common skin ailment which causes pimples

Actigall – also known as "Ursodiol" is a cholesterol medication used to dissolve gallstones

Antacids – a substance which neutralizes stomach acids

Benadryl – is commonly referred to as a Diphenhydramine which is an antihistamine used to treat allergies, hives and severe allergic reactions

Bilirubin – is a brownish yellow substance found in bile, it's produced when the liver breaks down old red blood cells.

BMI – short for "body mass index"

Bougie – a thin flexible surgical instrument used for exploring or dilating a passage of the body

Calcium – a mineral necessary for promoting stronger healthier bones and teeth

Carbs – short for "carbohydrates"

Dumping Syndrome - occurs when ingested foods bypass the stomach very rapidly and enter the small intestine largely undigested

Electrolytes – a substance that produces an electrically charged solution when dissolved in water

Glossary of Terms continued...

Endoscopy - a nonsurgical procedure used to examine a person's digestive tract using an endoscope

Gallstones - a hardened deposit within the fluid of the gallbladder

Gastric Band - is a silicone device placed around the upper section of the stomach, creating a small pouch above the band and thereby restricting the amount of food that can be comfortably eaten

Gastric Bypass - refers to a surgical procedure in which the stomach is divided into a small upper pouch and a much larger lower "remnant" pouch and then the small intestine is rearranged to connect to both.

Gastric Sleeve - is a surgical weight loss procedure in which the stomach is reduced to about 25% of its original size, by surgical removal of a large portion of the stomach along the greater curvature.

Gastritis - is an inflammation, irritation, or erosion of the stomach lining

GERD – short for "Gastroesophageal reflux disease"

GI Tract – short for "gastrointestinal tract" is an irritation, or erosion of the lining of the stomach

Hemoglobin - is the protein molecule in red blood cells that carries oxygen from the lungs to the body's tissues and returns carbon dioxide from the tissues back to the lungs.

Hives – a skin irritation caused by an allergic reaction

Incision - a surgical cut made in skin or flesh.

Glossary of Terms continued...

Invasive - involving entry into the living body (as by incision or by insertion of an instrument)

Intestines - are a long, continuous tube running from the stomach to the anus.

Isopure – is a brand of lactose free 100% whey protein

Malabsorption - is a state arising from abnormality in absorption of food nutrients across the GI tract.

Malnutrition - is a condition that results from eating a diet in which nutrients are not enough which then causes health problems.

Metabolism - is a term that is used to describe all chemical reactions involved in maintaining the living state of the cells and the organism.

Nexium – is a brand of PPI's that reduce stomach acid

NSAIDS – short for "Nonsteroidal anti-inflammatory drugs" such as aspirin, ibuprofen, naproxen

Nutrients - are components in foods that an organism uses to survive and grow.

Omeprazole – generic name of a PPI medication commercially known as Prilosec

OTC – short for "over the counter" medication

PCP - short for "primary care physician"

Platelet – are a component of blood whose function is to stop bleeding by clumping and clotting blood vessel injuries

Glossary of Terms continued...

PPI – short for "proton pump inhibitor"

TSH – short for "thyroid stimulating hormone" which is a pituitary hormone that stimulates the thyroid gland

Visceral Fat – is body fat that is stored within the abdominal cavity

VSG – short for "vertical sleeve gastrectomy"

Zantac – commercial name for ranitidine, an acid blocker.

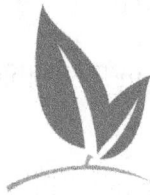

About The Authors

Dr. Guillermo Alvarez, a premier bariatric surgeon located in Piedras Negras, Coahuila, Mexico who is passionate about helping people fulfill their lifelong desire of attaining better health and a more fulfilling lifestyle. Dr. Alvarez has helped over 10,000 patients gain a new lease on life with the help of the gastric sleeve surgery.

Dr. Alvarez dedicates his practice to helping his patients achieve dramatic weight loss that leads to a healthier, longer and more prosperous life. Following weight loss surgery, many of Dr. Alvarez's patients are soon able to enjoy the benefits and joys of life that they previously could not while suffering from obesity. An improved love life, a more active lifestyle and the ability to enjoy quality time with friends and family are just some of the few positive changes that you will experience after weight loss surgery.

Rob Anspach, an author, speaker and business strategist located in Lancaster County, Pennsylvania, USA who is passionate about changing lives. Mr. Anspach serves as the Coordinator for The Endobariatric Foundation, and the Founder of Anspach Media.

Mr. Anspach is also the author of "Social Media Debunked", "Share: 27 Ways To Boost Your Social Media Experience, Build Trust and Attract Followers", "Optimize This: How Two Carpet Cleaners Consistently Beat Web Designers On The Search Engines" and "Lessons From The Dojo: 101 Ways To Improve Your Life, Business and Relationships".

Endobariatric

Dr. Alvarez's bariatric surgery Mexico facility is updated frequently to stay ahead of the normal standards used in the USA. The operating room is equipped with an emergency power plant that guarantees continuous electrical supply in case of an emergency such as an uncommon blackout. The hospital has a wide variety of diagnostic equipment that is found in large hospitals in the States, such as an MRI, Helicoidal CT Scan, Doppler Sonogram, etc.

This hospital has the top intensive care unit in this region with a staff of doctors and nurses that specialize in any trauma or emergency to support our patients in any case needed. You can feel safe in knowing that the staff of this facility is more than capable in handling your needs as a patient. The hospital is considered a "Specialized" hospital to handle the most difficult individual cases that are present.

The hospital includes 35 private rooms for patients and guest. Each room has telephone, TV, cable and a place for your guests to sleep. There are 4 suites available that also have a sofa and recliner.

The nursing staff is very professional and well trained for your care as a bariatric patient. There are 3 shifts (as opposed to the states - 2 shifts). We feel that is important that our entire team is fresh and alert to keep a 24-hour monitoring protocol. This entire staff is more than capable in handling all of your post-op care.

This hospital is a wonderful place for our bariatric patients to experience a safe and calm atmosphere and an excellent outcome during your recovery period. If you are considering this surgery for yourself or a family member, feel free to contact us any time. This is an option that will ensure you the best care from an excellent team of surgeons, nurses and top-notch hospital. We will be happy to have one of our coordinators assist you with more information and pricing.

1(866)697-5338 www.Endobariatric.com

Endo-Foundation

The Endobariatric Foundation is dedicated to helping those who truly desire to have the gastric sleeve procedure done, but might not have all the funds available to do so.

The ultimate goal of the foundation is to help those who are struggling financially avoid making the mistake of choosing a cheap gastric sleeve surgeon because they didn't have enough money.

"Money should never be that speed bump that slows you down and prevents you from improving your life".

So here's what we are doing to insure the success of the Foundation and make sure there are resources available when patients apply. We are setting aside a portion of every bill from every paying client and using it to fund this very worthwhile endeavor. This will be part of the Endobariatric legacy and will mean so much to so many.

To apply for a Foundation grant to help with your gastric sleeve surgery visit **www.Endobariatric.com/Endo-Foundation** today.

Become a Sponsor!

If you like to help people as much as we do, we invite you to become a sponsor. It can be a simple onetime gift of $25 or you can sponsor every month for whatever amount you deem life changing.

Mail your sponsorship monies to:

Endobariatric, SC
P.O. Box 6529 Eagle Pass TX 78853

Endo-Spa

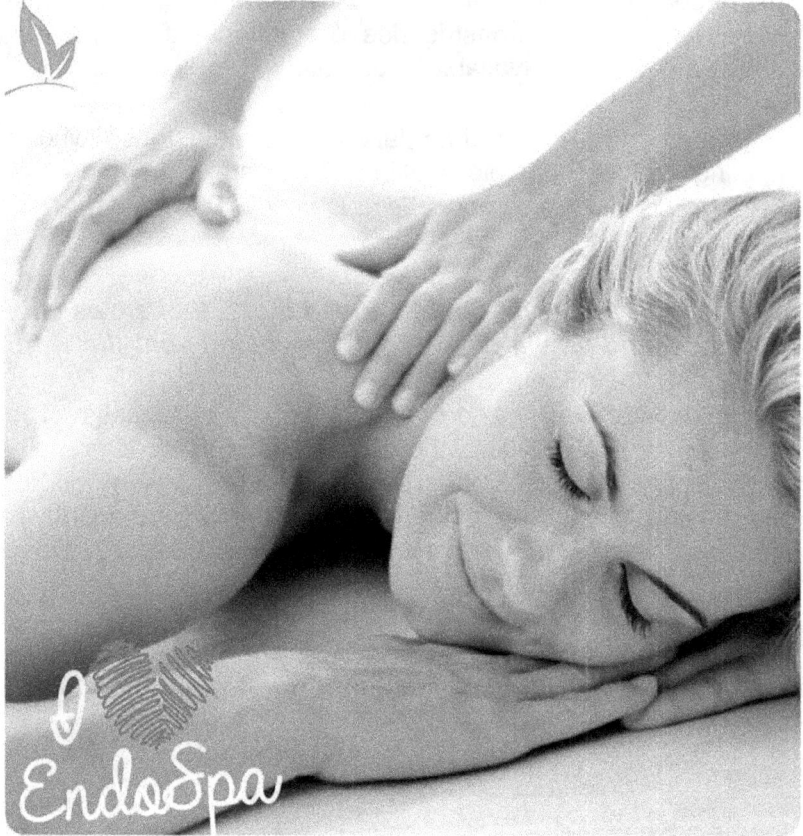

With relaxing surroundings, innovative treatments and a talented staff, EndoSpa nurtures your body, invigorates your senses and relaxes your mind. EndoSpa offers a wide array of spa treatments for men and women.

Massage – Facials – Laser Treatment

Hair Removal – Acoustic Wave Therapy

www.EndoSpa.mx

Endo-Store

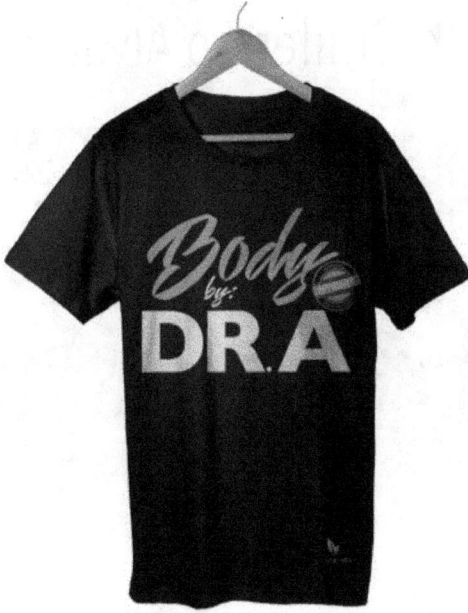

- Shirts
- Hats
- Bags
- Bottles
- Pillows
- Books
  And more!

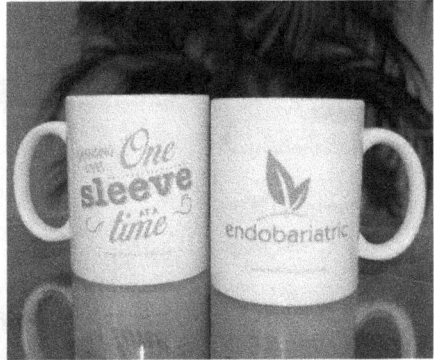

www.EndoStoreOnline.com

Other Books By The Authors

Dr. Guillermo Alvarez

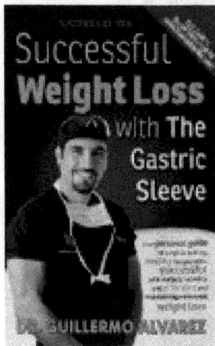

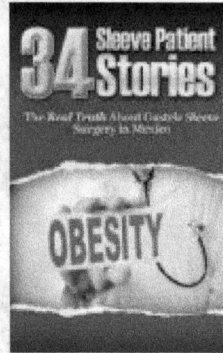

Rob Anspach

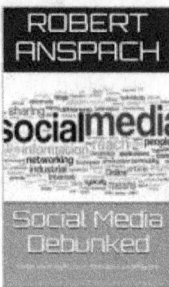

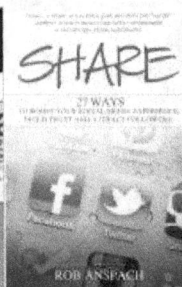

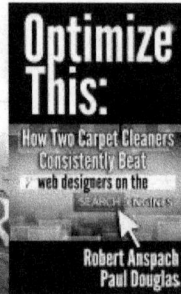

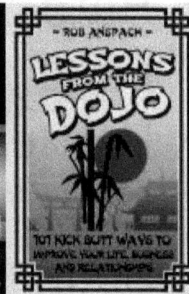

Available on Amazon

Be A Fan!

Follow Dr. Alvarez
on these Social Networks.

Facebook - www.facebook.com/endobariatric

Google+ - https://plus.google.com/+Endobariatric

Twitter - www.twitter.com/endobariatric

Pinterest - www.pinterest.com/endobariatric

Instagram - www.instagram.com/endobariatric

LinkedIn - www.linkedin.com/in/endobariatric

YouTube - www.youtube.com/endobariatric

Snapchat - www.snapchat.com/add/gmoalvarez

If you have a question and would like to get it answered...post it to Facebook, Twitter, Instagram or YouTube with the hashtag #AskDrA

Or send your question via Snapchat.

We might even answer it on our weekly show or in the next book.

Share This Book!

I mean it!

Tell your friends all about this book.

Share where you bought it.

Share it at lunch!

Share it at the gym!

Share it on the beach!

Share it on social media.

Share it using this hashtag...

TheAskDrABook

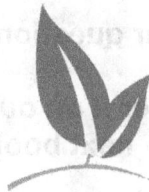

www.ingramcontent.com/pod-product-compliance
Lightning Source LLC
Chambersburg PA
CBHW070254290326
41930CB00041B/2520